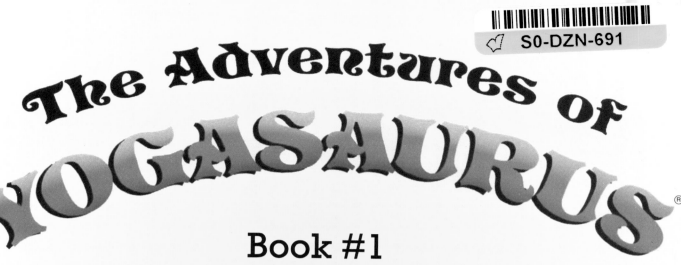

The Adventures of YOGASAURUS

Book #1
Yogasaurus Makes a Friend
by
Kenneth E. Duncan

Illustrated by John Steven Gurney

www.yogasaurus.com

My special thanks to Susan "Betsy" Light and JSG.

Always consult with your physician or health professional
before performing any new exercise program.

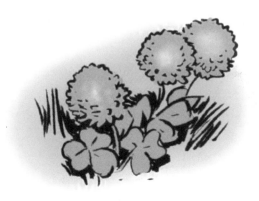

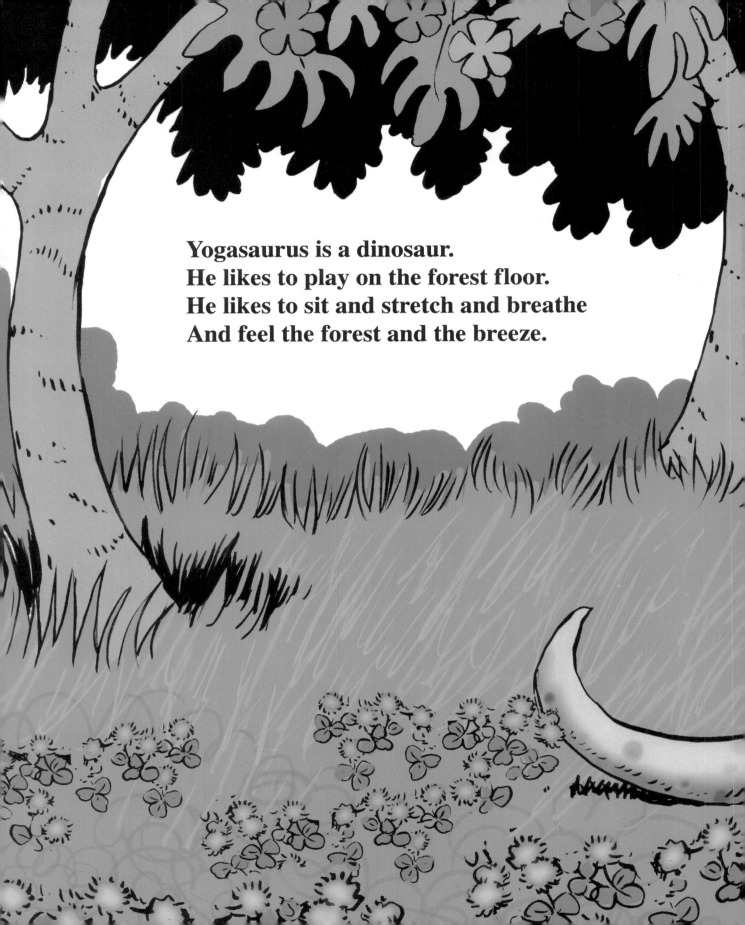

Yogasaurus is a dinosaur.
He likes to play on the forest floor.
He likes to sit and stretch and breathe
And feel the forest and the breeze.

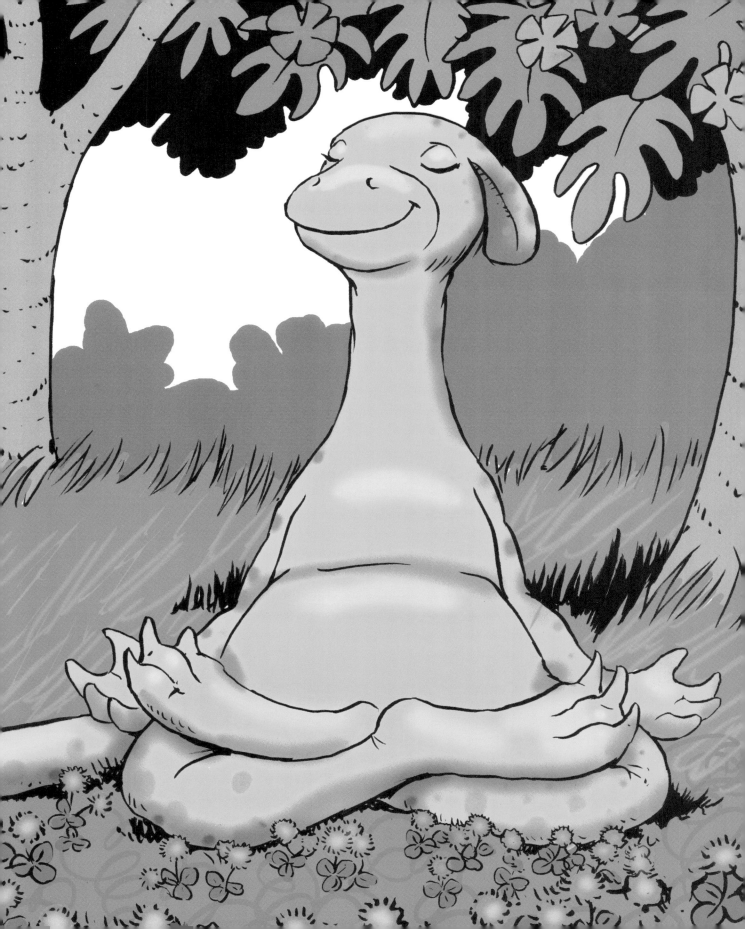

Especially in the clover green,
Because it is his favorite thing
To look at, and be with, and ponder the shapes
Of the flowers with petals colored like grapes.

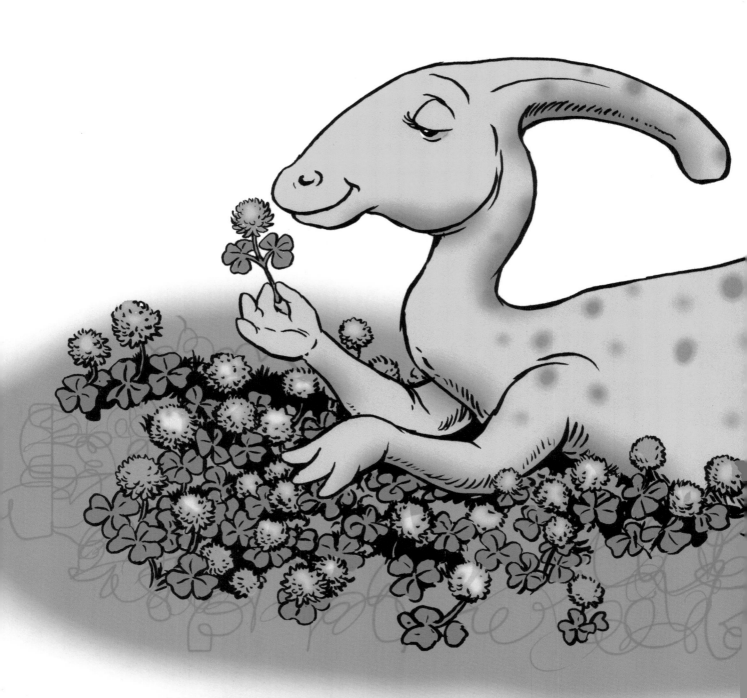

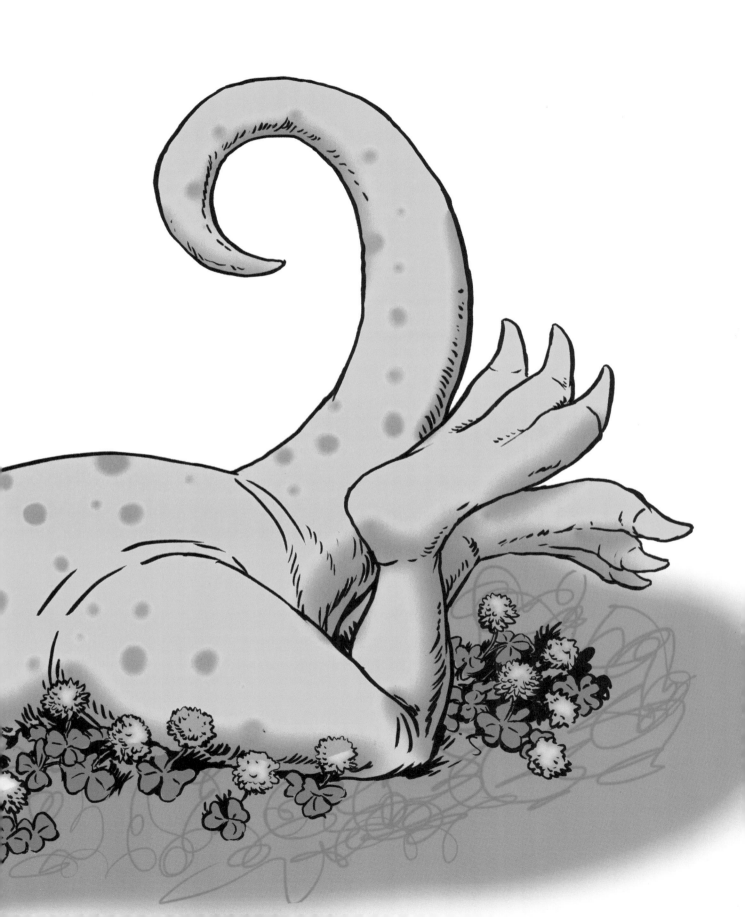

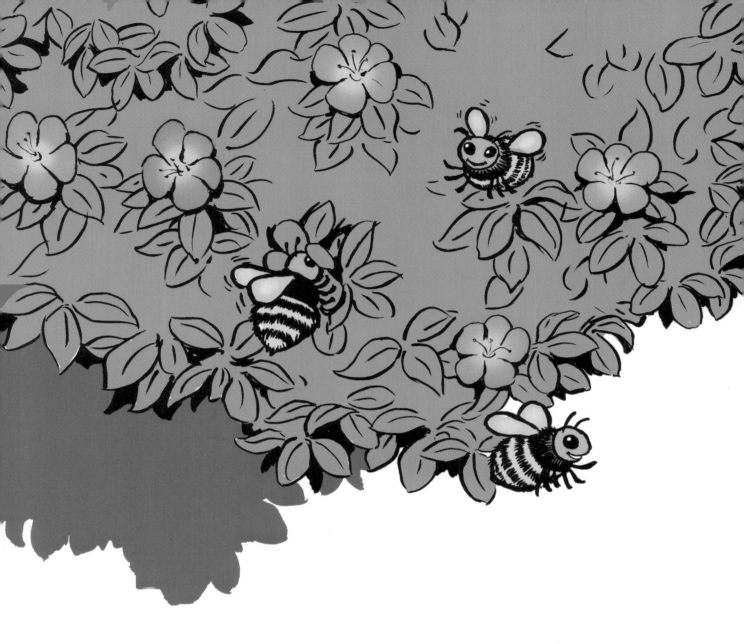

The flowers are fluffy like the bees
That buzz the flowers for nectar free.
Yogasaurus likes the bees and their bee-buzz sound.
He likes to watch them as he sits on the ground.

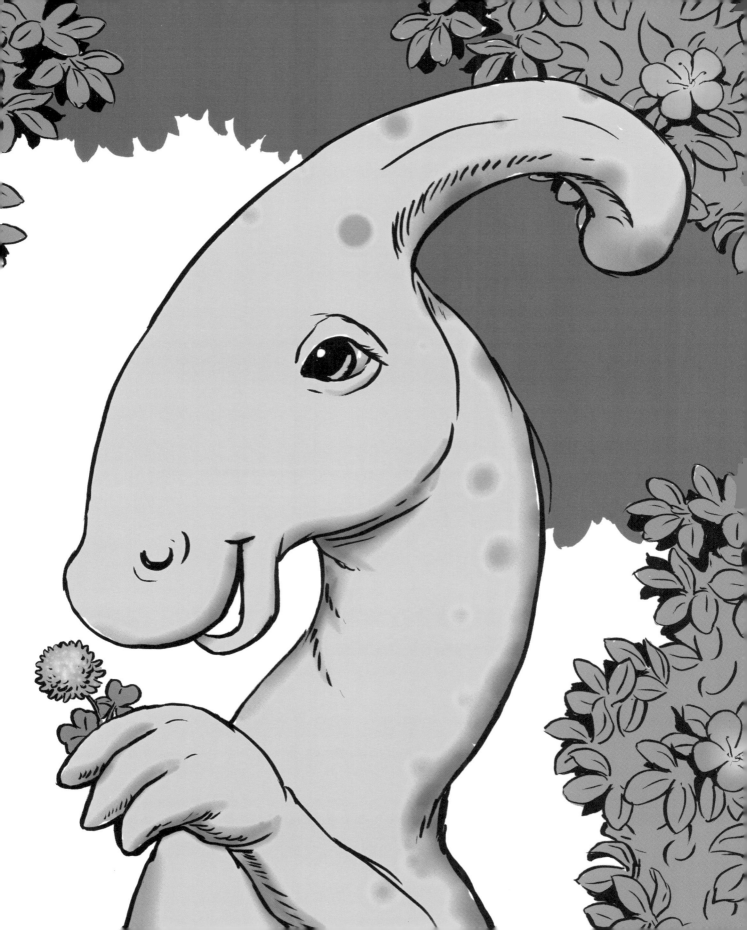

He watches dragonflies and butterflies
And wonders as they dart and flutter by.
He likes how they move around in the air,
Pretty and friendly, without a care.

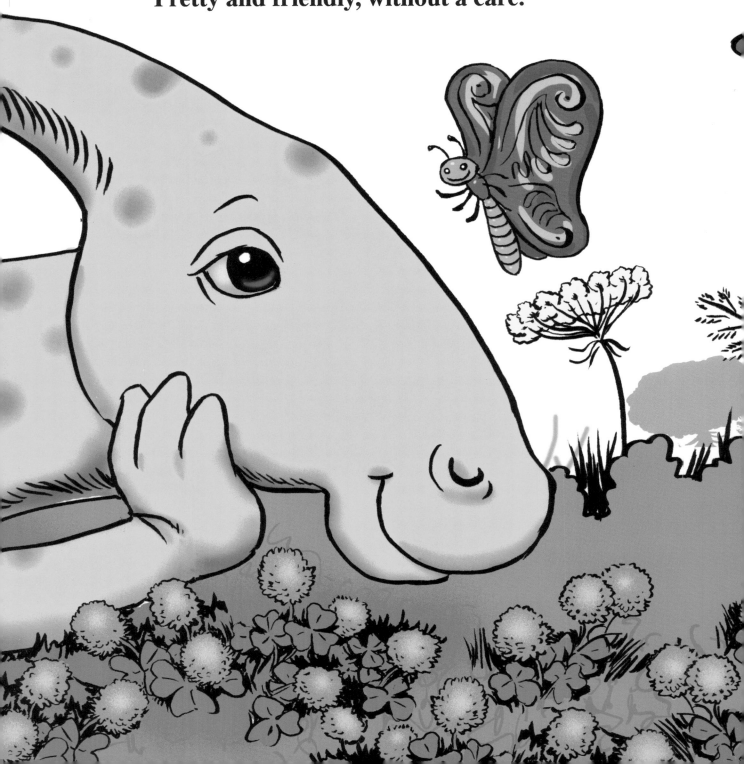

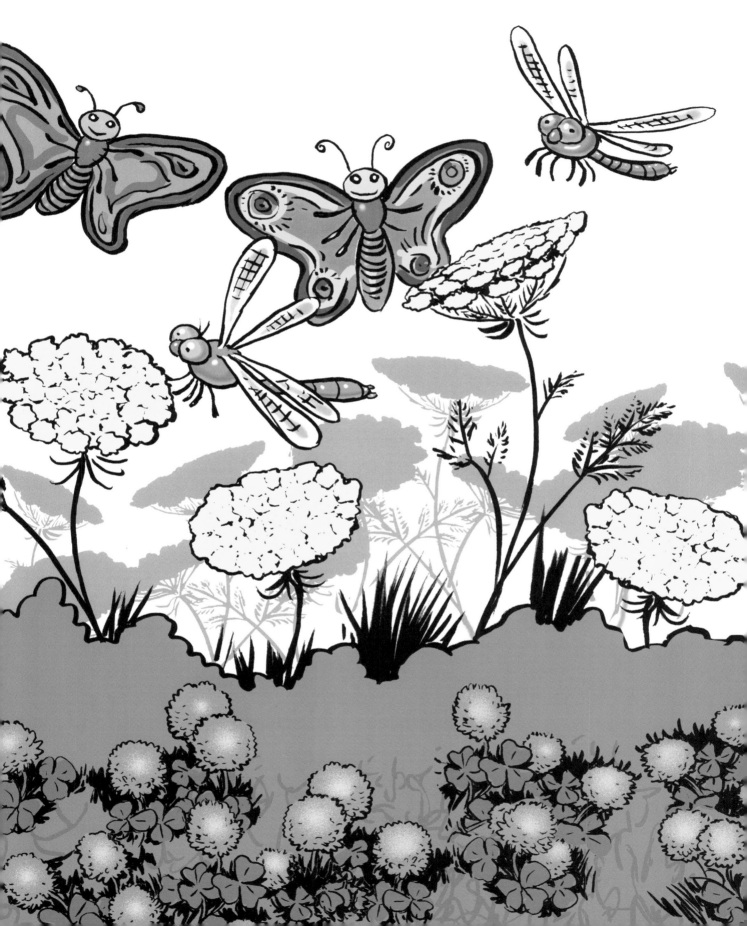

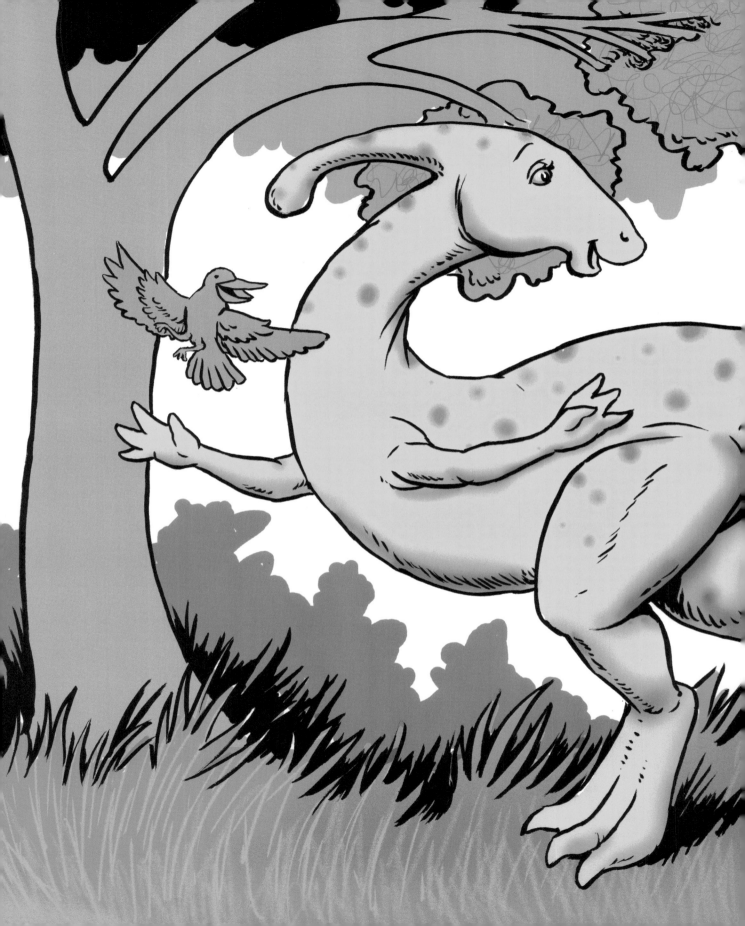

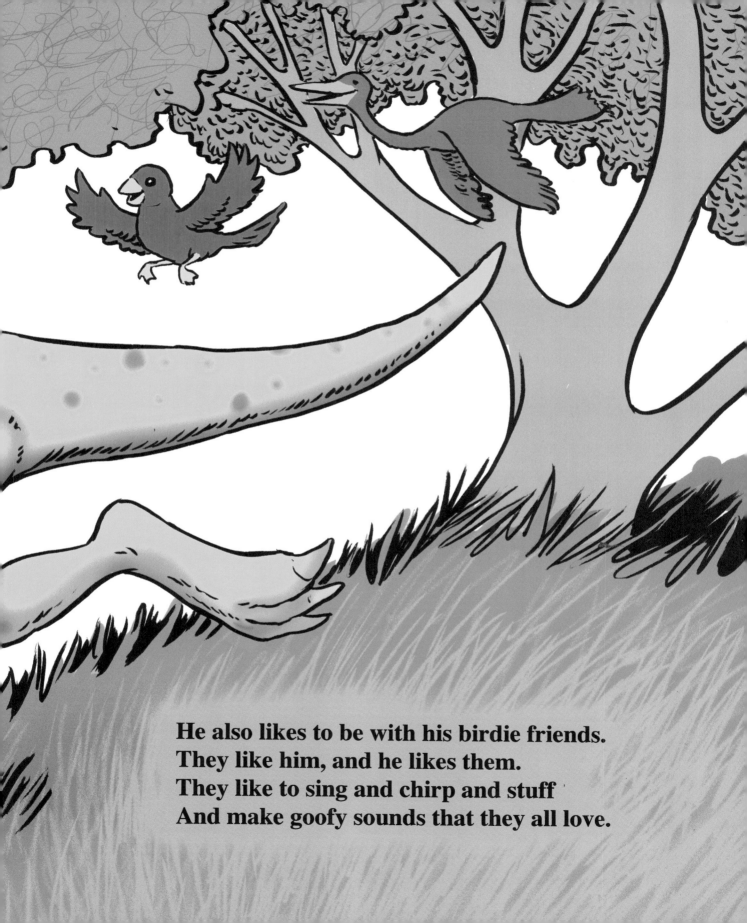

He also likes to be with his birdie friends.
They like him, and he likes them.
They like to sing and chirp and stuff
And make goofy sounds that they all love.

They like to hang out and have fun and play
And bend and stretch and breathe all day.

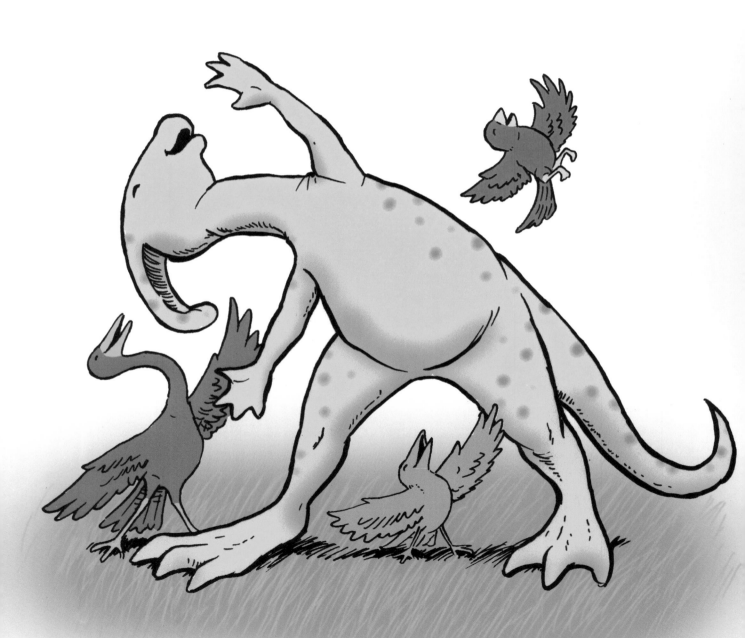

They would sing and dance and joke together
And make up stories in all kinds of weather.

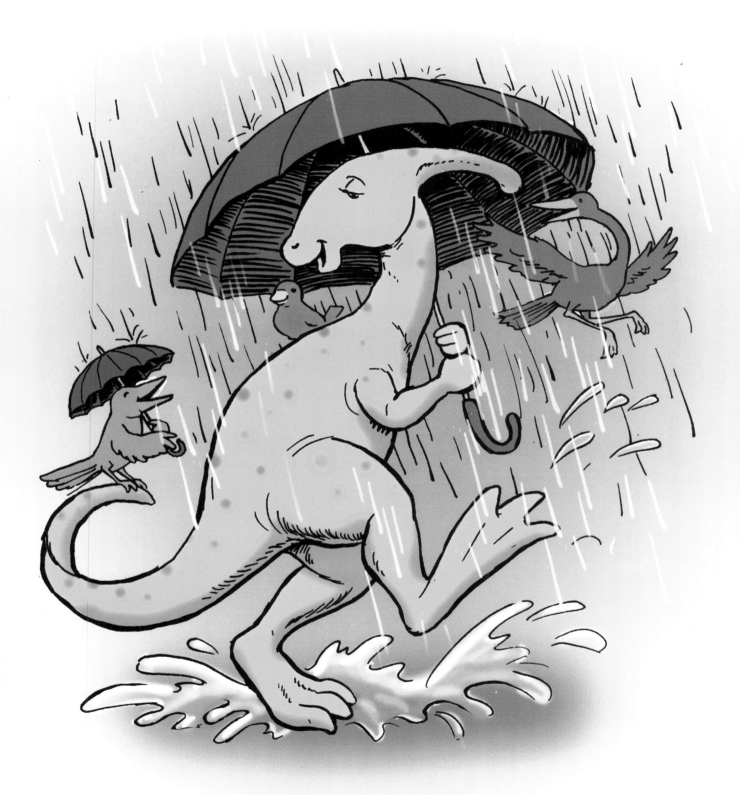

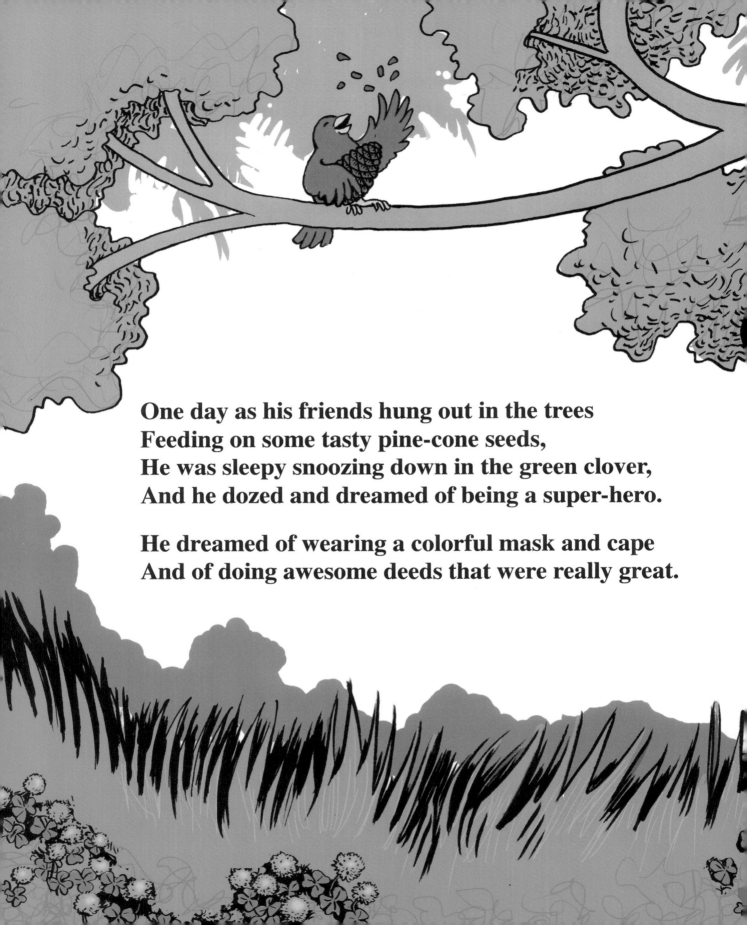

One day as his friends hung out in the trees
Feeding on some tasty pine-cone seeds,
He was sleepy snoozing down in the green clover,
And he dozed and dreamed of being a super-hero.

He dreamed of wearing a colorful mask and cape
And of doing awesome deeds that were really great.

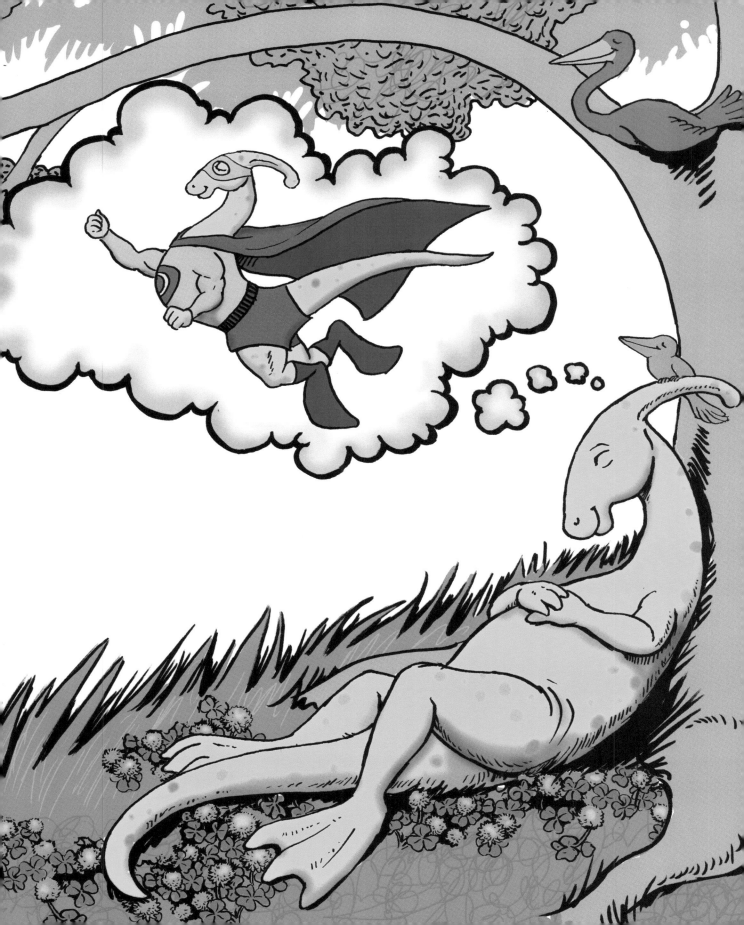

Then all of a sudden, as he was dreaming in his head
He actually was attacked by a Tyrannosaurus Rex!

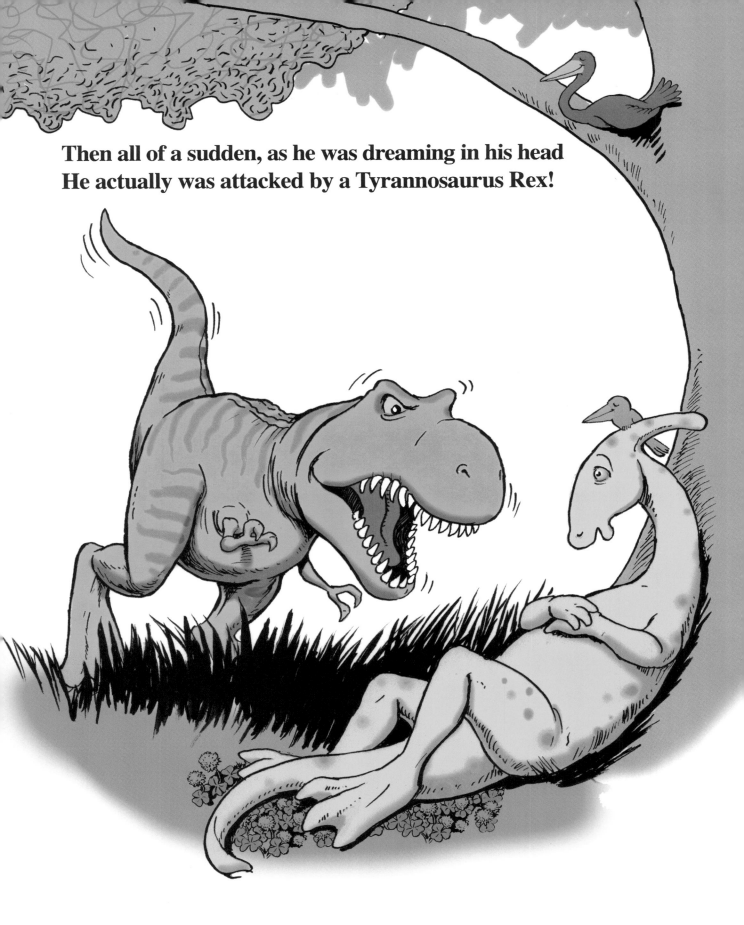

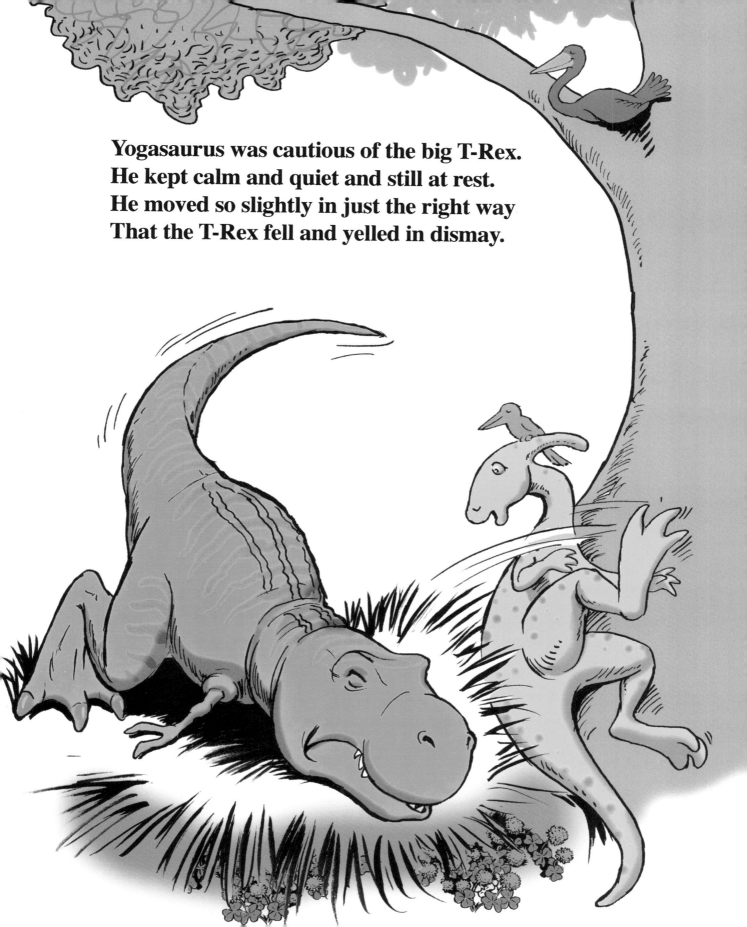

Yogasaurus was cautious of the big T-Rex.
He kept calm and quiet and still at rest.
He moved so slightly in just the right way
That the T-Rex fell and yelled in dismay.

T-Rex fell fast and onto the ground.
And let out a startling, loud and long sound.

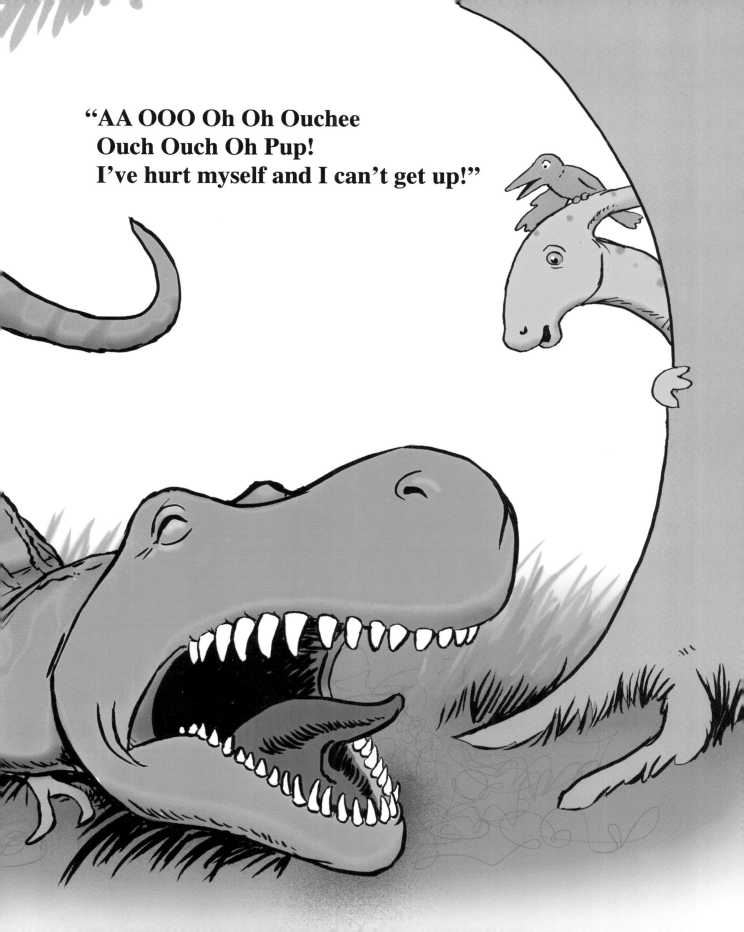

"AA OOO Oh Oh Ouchee
Ouch Ouch Oh Pup!
I've hurt myself and I can't get up!"

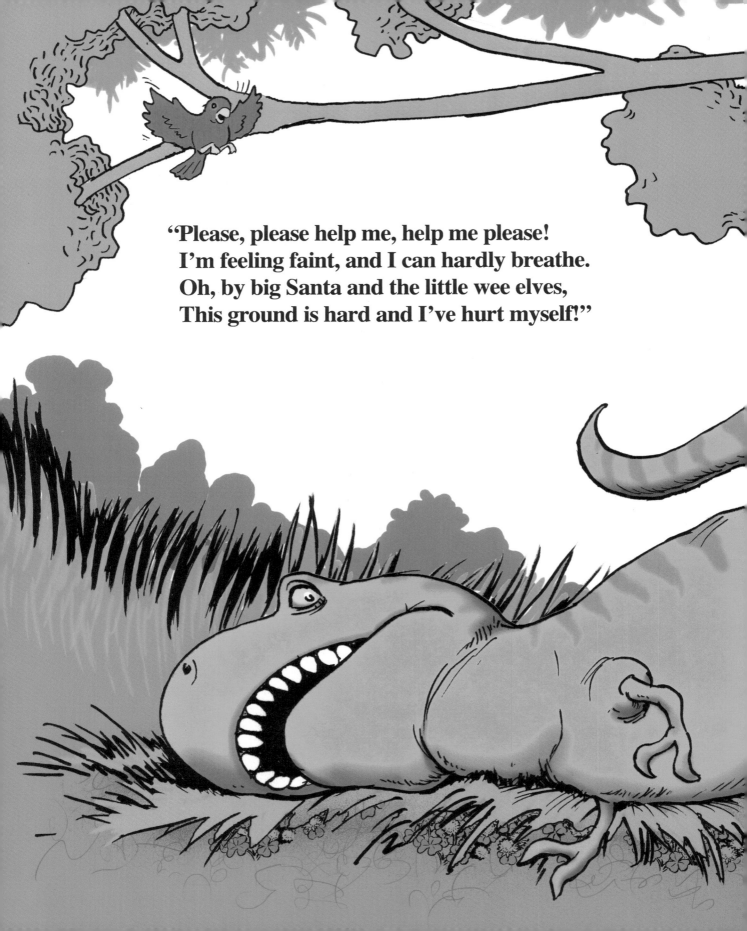

"Please, please help me, help me please!
I'm feeling faint, and I can hardly breathe.
Oh, by big Santa and the little wee elves,
This ground is hard and I've hurt myself!"

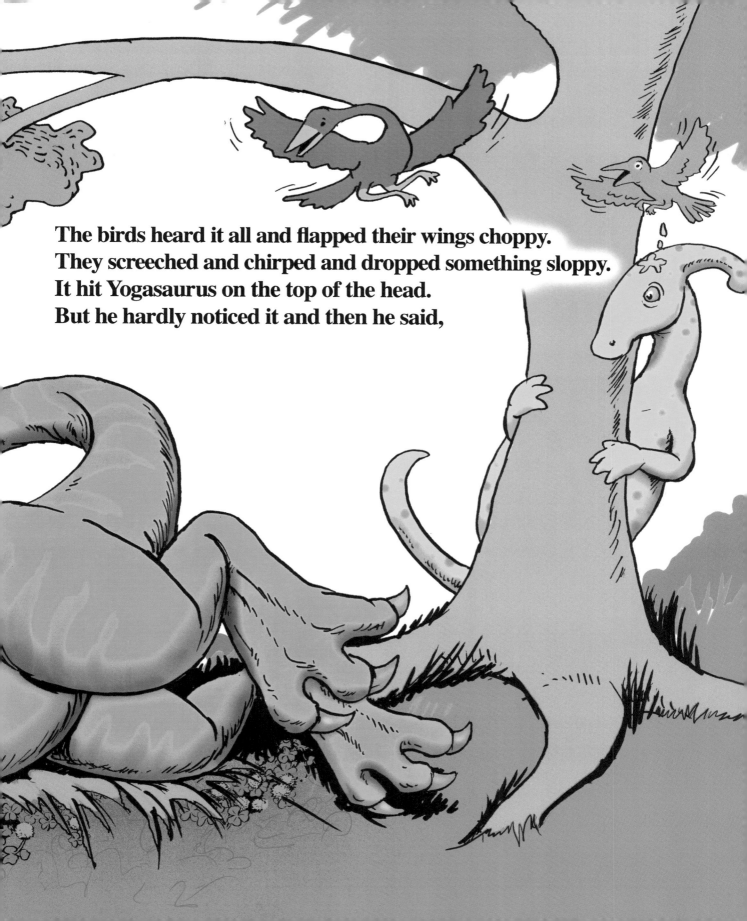

The birds heard it all and flapped their wings choppy.
They screeched and chirped and dropped something sloppy.
It hit Yogasaurus on the top of the head.
But he hardly noticed it and then he said,

"I'm Yogasaurus, and I'm curious now to see,
  If I help you, will you promise not to hurt me?"

"Oh yes. Oh, yes. I give you my promise indeed.
  I swear I won't claw you, bite or make you bleed."

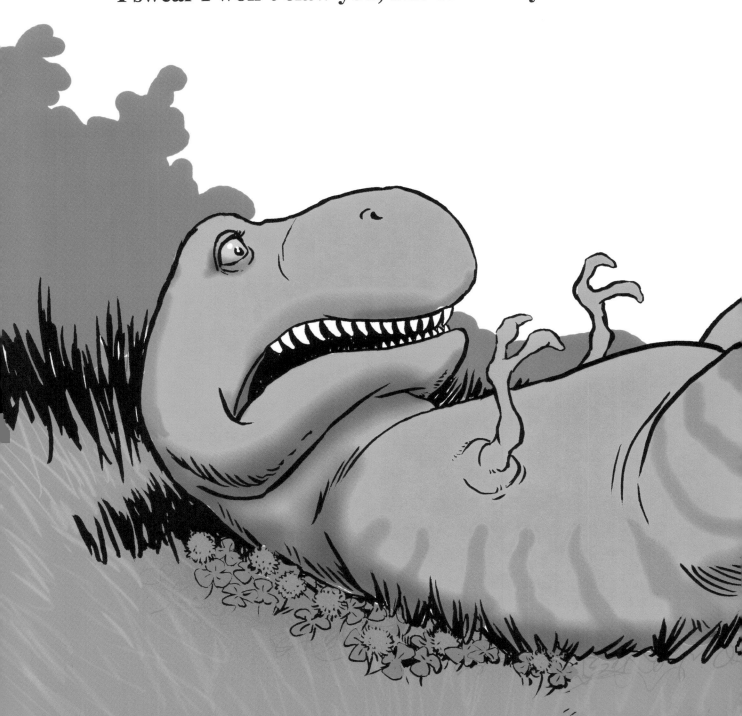

"Okay, then, Big-T, I'll take you at your word,
And I will help you feel better and not to hurt."

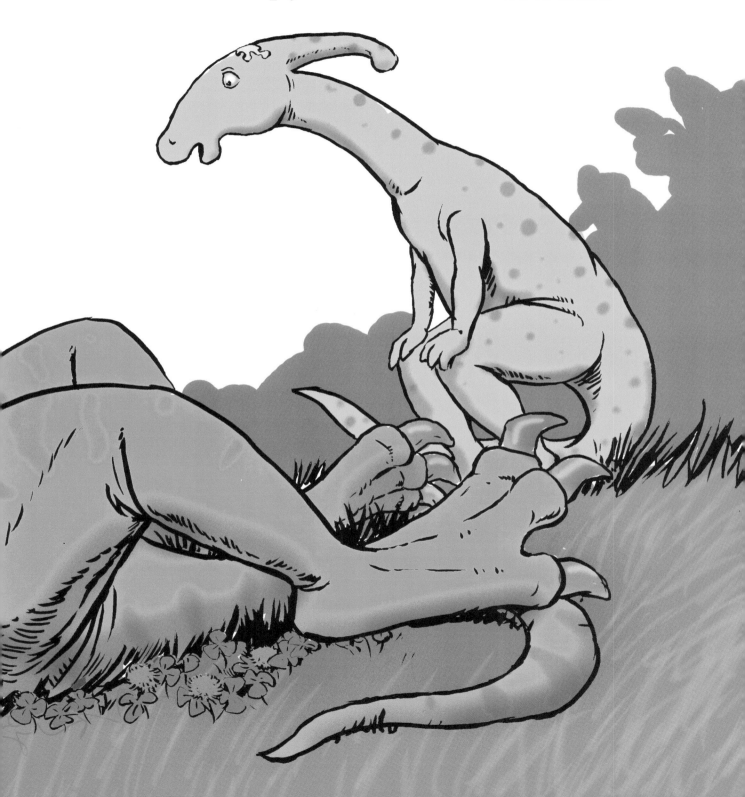

So Yogasaurus taught T-Rex to breathe easy in and out,
Nice and slowly through his nose and mouth.
In through the nose and then out the nose,
And vice-a-versa and so it goes.

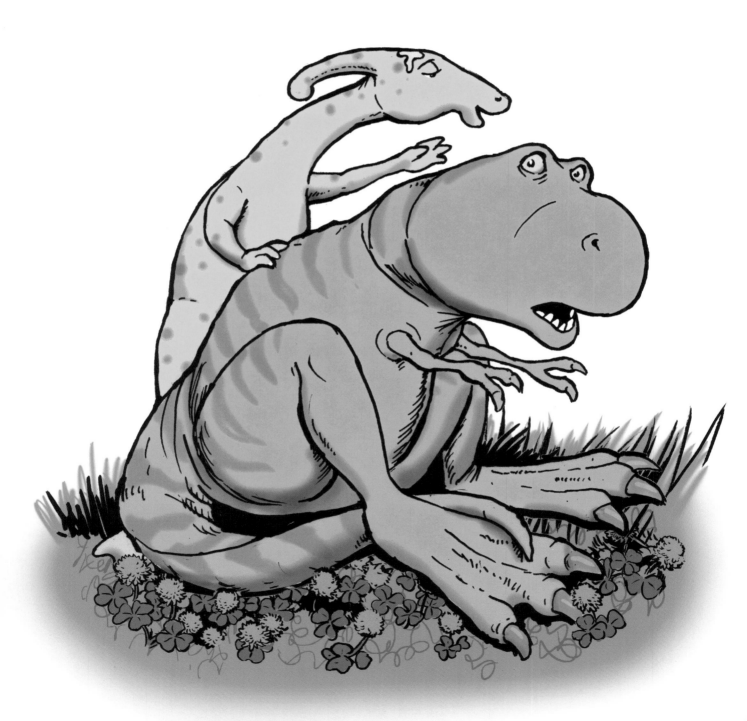

In through the nose and then out the mouth.
Pulling fresh air freely north and south.

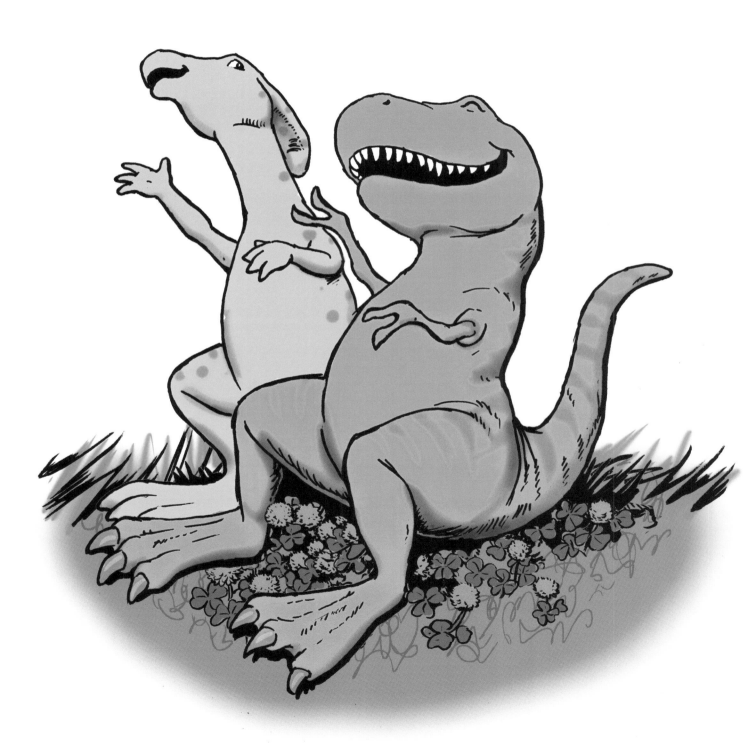

Then after a while, T-Rex calmed down
And he began not to wear such a frown.

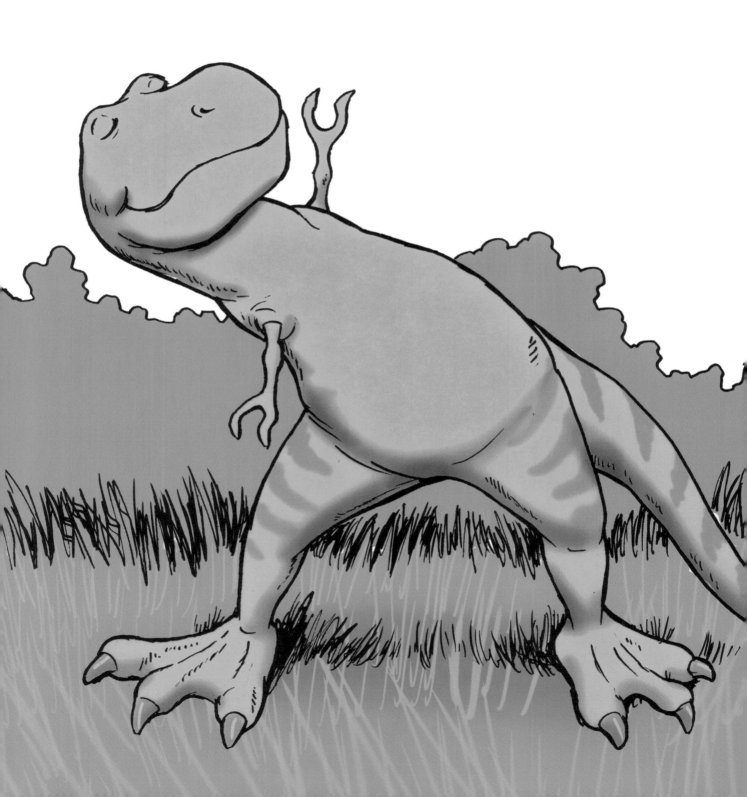

Because, as he relaxed and the pain went away,
The T-Rex began to feel better that very same day.

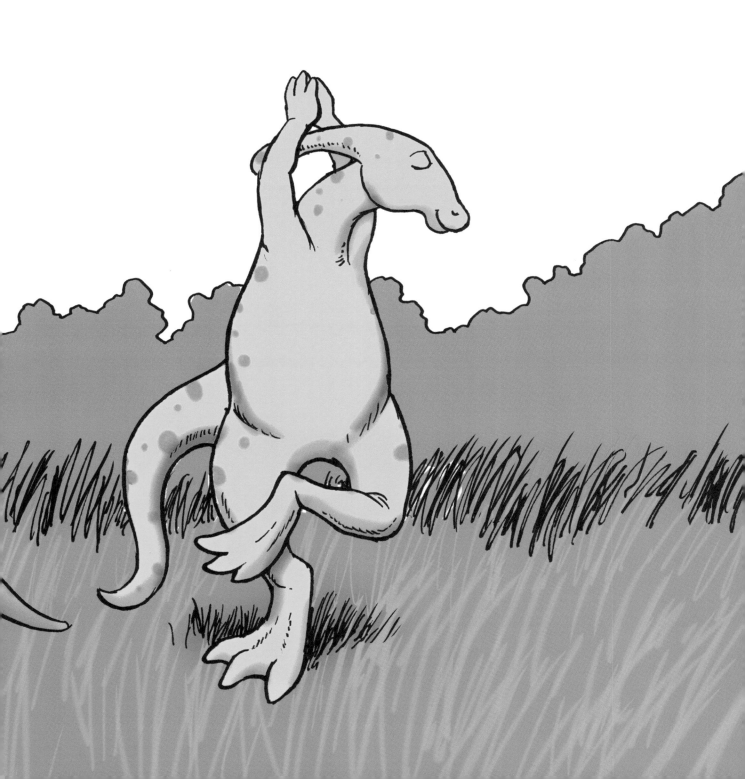

So Yogasaurus ended up liking T-Rex like a brother,
And they became good friends and helped one another.

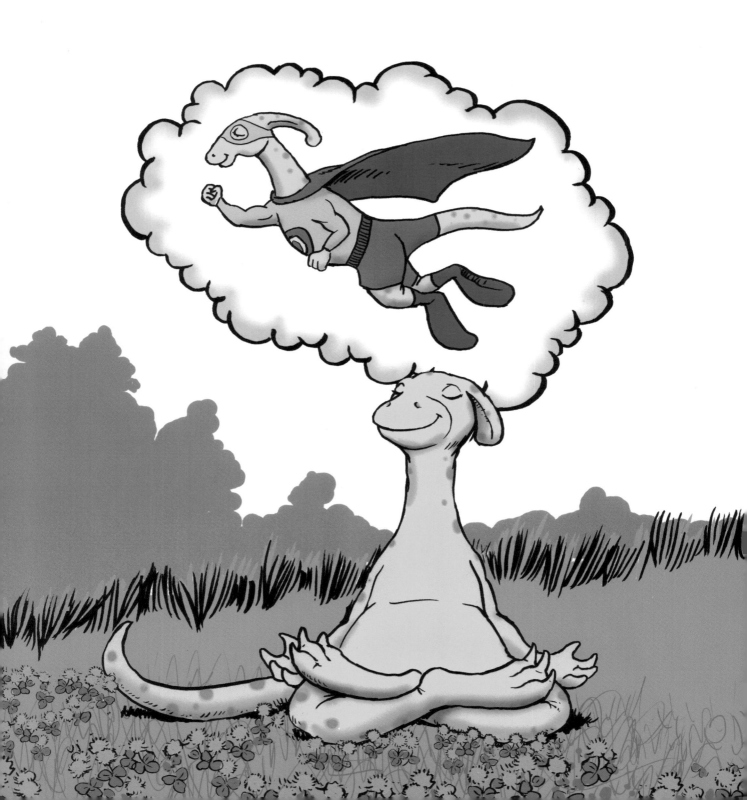

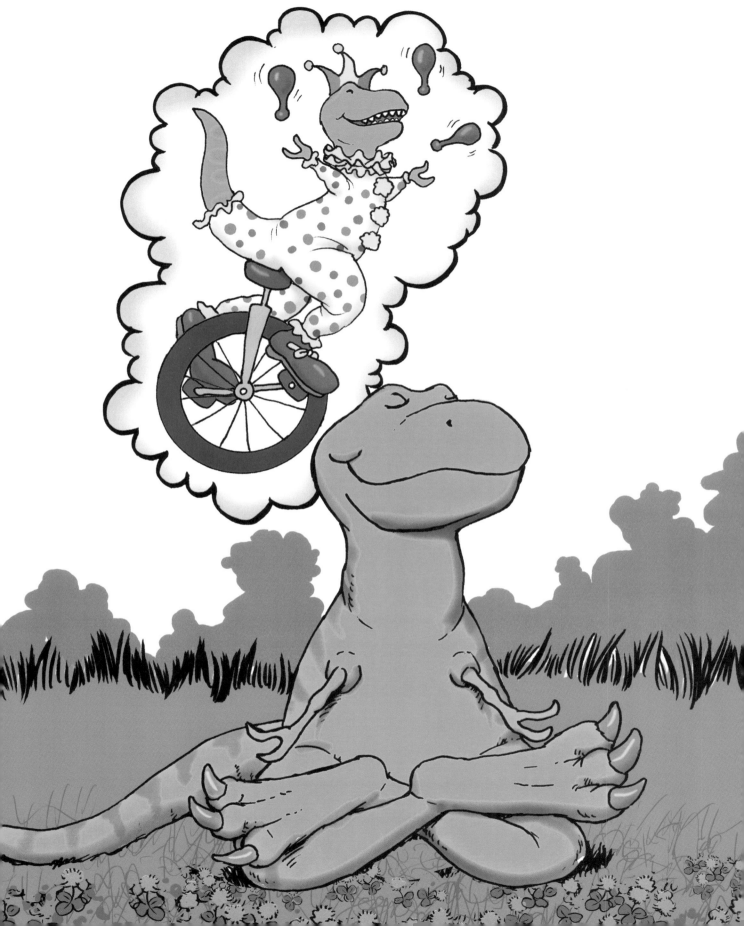

Later Yogasaurus taught the T-Rex to have fun stretching and breathing with the Salutation to the Sun.

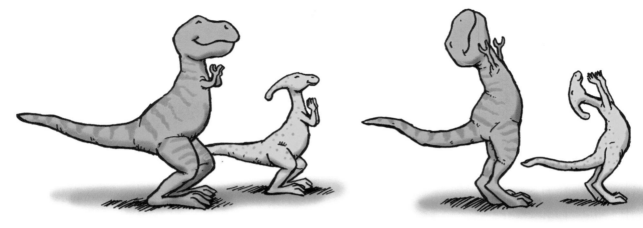

1. Stand in Mountain Pose

2. Inhale: Reach up

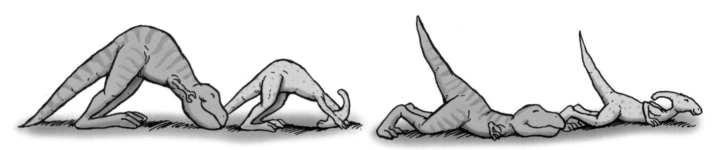

**5. Exhale:
Downward Facing Dog**

**6. Inhale into Plank
Exhale to the floor**

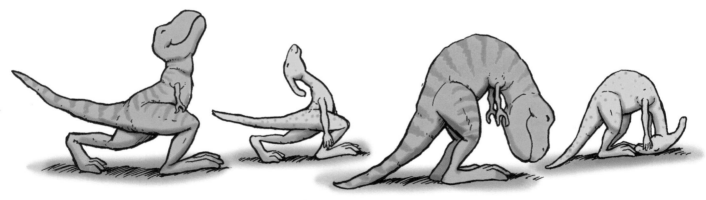

**9. Inhale: Step forward
with right foot into Lunge**

10. Exhale: Forward Bend

**Yogasaurus encourages his friend – and you – to be safe.
And not to push too hard or move at too quick a pace.**

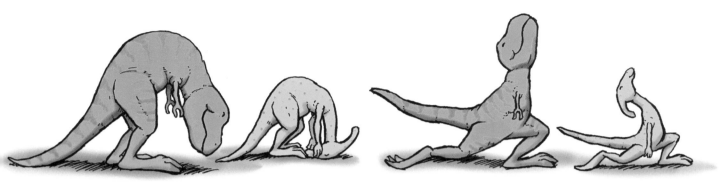

3. Exhale: Forward bend

4. Inhale: Step back with right foot into Lunge

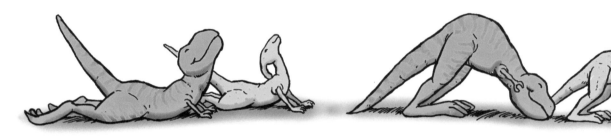

7. Inhale: Cobra

8. Exhale: Downward Facing Dog

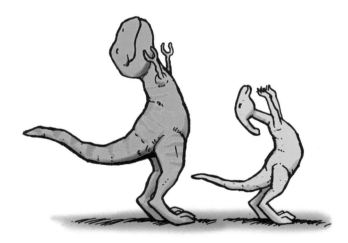

11. Inhale: Reach up

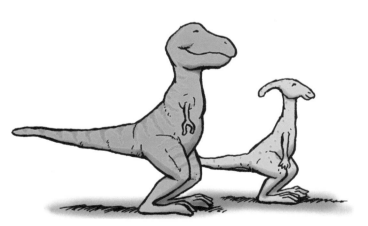

12. Exhale: Mountain Pose

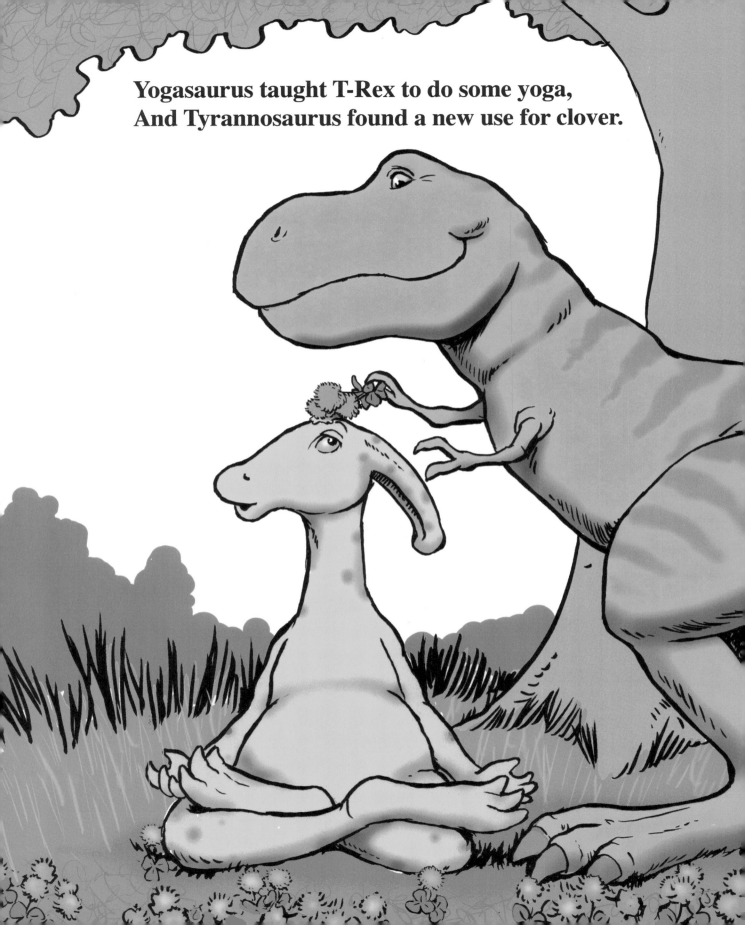

Yogasaurus taught T-Rex to do some yoga,
And Tyrannosaurus found a new use for clover.

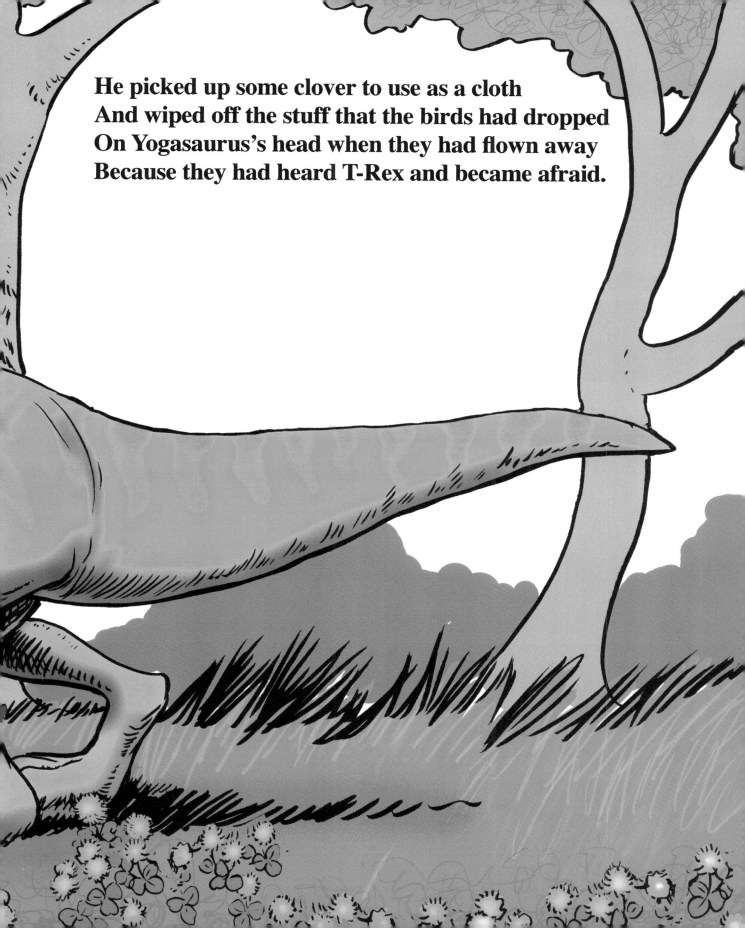

He picked up some clover to use as a cloth
And wiped off the stuff that the birds had dropped
On Yogasaurus's head when they had flown away
Because they had heard T-Rex and became afraid.

The birds apologized later, said it wasn't on purpose.
Yogasaurus laughed, said it wasn't the worstest
Thing that had ever happened to him,
But please try not to do it again.

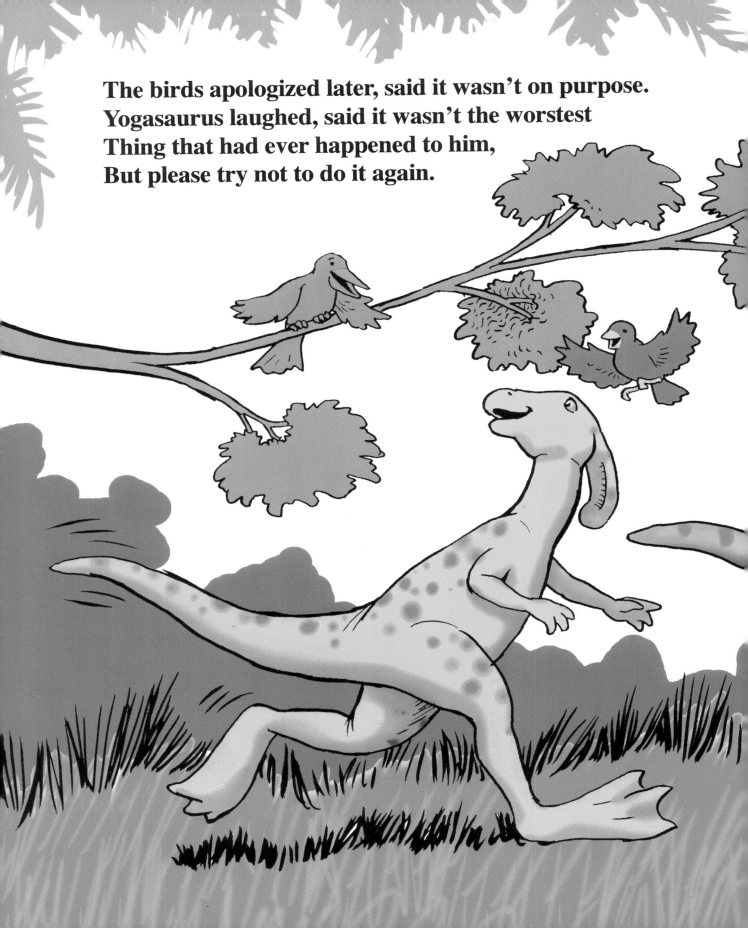

Then the friends were happy and not sad blue,
And they rolled and chortled about the air-born poo.
And they chatted and darted and ran and played,
And had tons of fun telling of that great day.

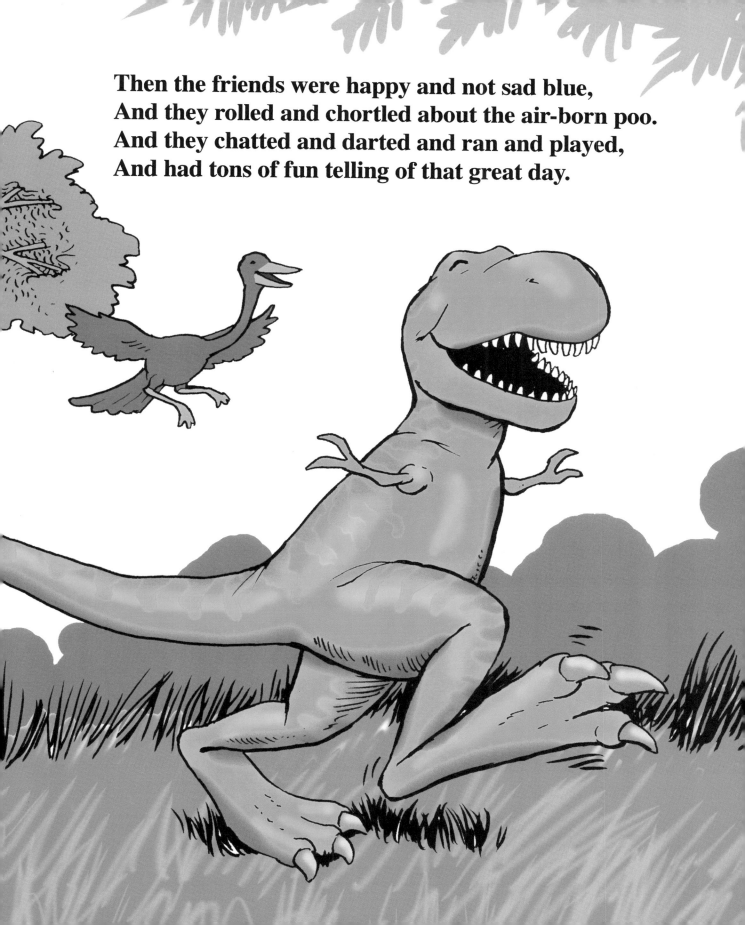

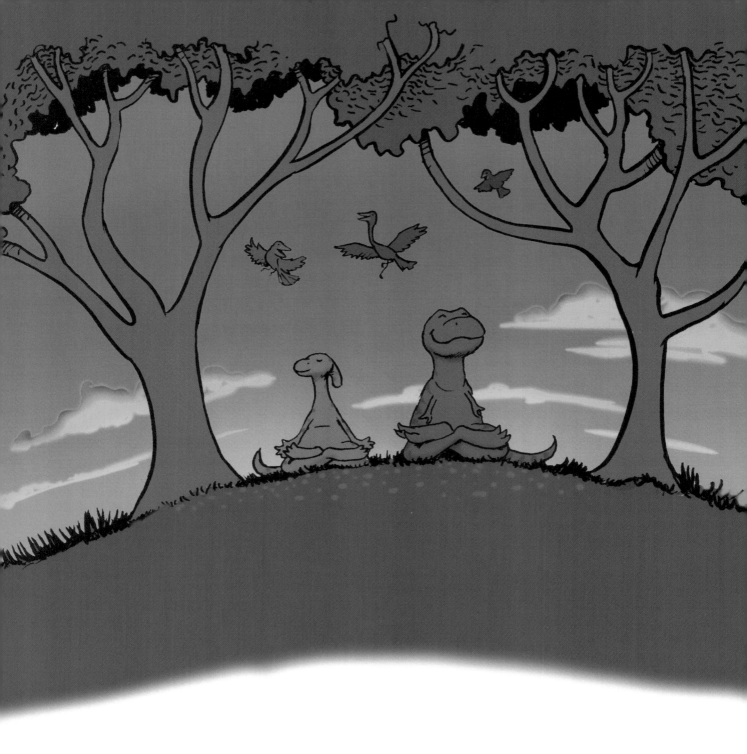

So for now we will say that our story is over,
And we will leave Yogasaurus and his friends in the clover.